CLEANSING

When, Why, What and How to Cleanse, for Everyone.

By Chris Hallford

CLEANSING WITH THE SEASONS Copyright © 2011 by Chris Hallford.
All rights reserved. Printed in the United States of America.
No part of this book may be used or reproduced or transmitted in any form or by any means, electronic or mechanical, including photocopying, recording, or by any information storage and retrieval system without the written permission from Chris Hallford, except for the inclusion of brief quotations in a review.

FIRST EDITION

Book Cover Design: Chris Hallford
Cover Image: iStockphoto
Chinese Symbols Art Work by Christian Noble - www.nobleartdesign.wordpress.com

Library of Congress Cataloging-in-Publication Data
Hallford, Chris
Cleansing with the Seasons
When, Why, What and How to Cleanse, for Everyone.
by Chris Hallford - 1st ed
Includes bibliographical references

ISBN # 978-0-9848739-1-3
$7.99 Soft cover

Please Note! The information in this book is from many sources, including modern medicine, ancient Chinese medicine, naturopathy, and the author's personal study, observation and experience. The conclusions expressed herein are those of the author's and are not to be taken as medical advice.

Cleansing with the Seasons is written and published as an information resource and educational guide for both professionals and non-professionals. It should not be used as a substitute for your physician's advice. Be sure to work with a physician who understands cleansing.

The author by no means is recommending you to follow the advice in this book without consulting your physician first and therefore assumes no responsibility for the misuse or application of the information in this book.

*this book is **dedicated to**
Tor-bjorn M. Hanson,
who taught me the wisdom of nature and the
potential of the human body*

Foreword

I believe that the books we need find us as much as we find them. If this gem of a book has found you, then count yourself lucky. Chris Hallford has written a beautifully succinct and timely book about detoxification.

We live in an age of rampant toxicity, and it is my opinion, and the opinion of thousands of other experts in the field of holistic medicine, that toxicity is the number one cause of the current epidemics of cancer and other chronic illness. But there is a solution; Chris outlines numerous easy-to-follow protocols to detoxify your body, and if you follow his advice you can be assured of health improvement.

In 20 years of treating thousands of patients I have seen these protocols working repeatedly. What is so refreshing about this book is how Chris integrates Eastern and Western approaches to detoxification. These integrated health improvement plans are quite do-able and there are many practical tips which clearly derive from the author's own experience.

I would add that the appendices alone are worth the price of the book! In these Chris has captured the essence of many breakthrough approaches to health improvement.

In summary this is a great guidebook on the journey to health recovery or for the maintenance of vibrant good health. Study it well and you will be assured of success. I will be carrying this book in my clinic and recommending it to my patients.

Adam Atman L.Ac. MMQ.

~ *Board Certified Acupuncturist*
~ *Director of Medical Qi Gong Clinic*
~ *Acupuncture College Instructor and Clinic Supervisor*
~ *Medical Herbalist*
~ *Medical Qi Gong Practitioner and Instructor*
~ *Founder of Sacred Acupuncture*

Chris' Story *(the quick version)*

A long journey through health problems has brought me to this book, and you. From a young age I was on antibiotics for ear infections and then later on for acne. Combine that with the massive amounts of drugs I took as a teenager for my low back pain, and you get total destruction of anything good in my digestive system, which is, of course, where over 80% of the body's immune system is found.

I suffered my entire childhood with food allergies, diarrhea, stomach pains and food poisoning incidences. In my teenage years I was stricken with severe low back pain, which brought me to a professional who practiced Chinese medicine and acupuncture. He eventually became my first professional mentor.

From a young age I was introduced to healing my pain and body through mental, emotional, spiritual and physical strategies based on the laws of the five elements and Chinese medicine.

Once I became a health professional and gained much more knowledge about the body and health, I began treating myself instinctually with cleanses and probiotics.

After many years of experimenting, I was able to finally eat foods I never thought I could eat again and increase my energy to a level that met my true potential.

The cleanses served as an elimination process for an entire life of toxin build up as well as a foundation to build up the good bacteria in my stomach and immune system again.

Couple all of that with my first true professional love, Eastern medicine and Chinese acupuncture, and you get a group of cleanses that align with the seasons and elements and are aimed at healing every dimension of the human body; mentally, emotionally, spiritually and physically.

Now my energy and health are abundant, and the rest is history.

Chris Hallford
www.hallfordhealth.com

Contents

1	Intro
2	How the Seasons Relate to Life
6	When, Why, What and How to Cleanse, for Everyone
27	Spring Cleanse
35	Summer Cleanse
44	Autumn Cleanse
51	Winter Cleanse
59	Earth Cleanse
63	Off-Season Nutrition

Appendix

66	Cleanse Options List
69	Food Combining and Layering
75	Antioxidants
76	Allergy Foods
77	Cooking and Eating Rules
80	Primary Nutrition

86	Super Alkalizers
89	Inflammation Fighters
91	The No-No list
95	Unrefined vs. Refined Carbs
98	Master Cleanse Recipe
99	Pysillium Husk Mixture
100	Yin Yang Foods
101	Coconut Oil
102	80/20 Rules
103	Blood Type Foods
104	Bibliography

INTRO

I was considering not doing an intro, because who really reads an intro? But I realized that this book serves a purpose for me beyond cleansing.

I really wish that many people were still alive in my life right now. My mom, many clients and friends, the list is unfortunately long of people in my life who have passed away WAY too early from cancer and disease.

If you are reading this intro, than I hope it inspires you to cradle your health with both arms and nurture it in a way that makes disease and cancer succumb to your powers.

If there is one simple way to do that, it is through periodic cleansing. No matter what your history is, the body is so powerful, so self-correcting that all you need to do is create some space for it to heal, and it will do the rest.

Disease and cancer enter the body via mental, emotional, spiritual and physical traumas that we do not deal with. This book is a tool for dealing with these traumas.

How the Seasons Relate to Life

Everyone knows that nature is something we all should model after as often as possible, especially if health is on our agenda. What if I were to tell you that every result or goal you want in life follows the cycles of the four seasons?

Without writing an entire book on the subject, here is a very simple outline of how the seasons work together with the five elements and your inner workings. While there are four main seasons and five elements (Fire, Earth, Metal, Water and Wood), the element of Earth coincides with a fifth season. This fifth season encompasses all seasons and is the transition period between each. It is the element that nurtures all others and is a short period of time with the most energy. More will be explained within each seasonal cleanse.

This is an interpretation of the laws of nature and how to use them for creating goals and success in one's life. They are based on Chinese medicine, acupuncture, and the teachings of my first professional mentor, Tor-bjorn M. Hanson.

Spring (**Wood**)

Sowing, dreaming, cleansing, fertilizing, planting, goal setting, responsibility, forgiving, letting go, deciding, beginning, and assertiveness.

Summer (**Fire**)

Blossoming, flourishing, watering, weeding, following through, optimism, enthusiasm, focusing, concentrating, anticipating success, enjoying, continuing, and joy.

Autumn (**Metal**)

Harvesting, reaping, realizing, receiving, acceptance, understanding, calmness, discipline, completing, finishing, and compassion.

Winter (**Water**)

Rest, reflection, storing, conserving, appreciating, gratitude, ambition, modest, honest, will power, evaluating, and cautiousness.

What does this mean? Well, think of an idea or goal; let's say "lose weight." Now watch it go through the four seasons (also imagine a farmer going through a similar process with their crops through the seasons).

Spring

- Plant seeds (set goal - how much weight, when to reach goal by, etc.) and start a new beginning.
- One must let go of certain ideas, bad influences (people and addictions) and issues to move on to achieve this goal.
- One must forgive their self for failing (to lose weight) in the past (if applicable).
- One must be assertive in their actions for this goal to take flight and gain momentum.

Summer

- One must follow through with their spring ideas and concentrate on enjoying the process.
- One must water (reinforce) ideas and plan by consistently focusing on what is right and weeding out the bad thoughts and influences (obstacles) that pop up and try to prevent one from achieving their goal.
- Anticipating success is essential to maintaining motivation and joy.

Autumn

- This is where one obtains their goal.
- They have realized their dream and harvested it.
- One reaps all the benefits/fruits of their hard work now and has compassion for the entire process.

Winter

- Now is the time to reflect on achievement and figure out 1) what worked? 2) what didn't work? and 3) what can you do differently next time?
- One takes time to appreciate their efforts and results while being cautious not to be reckless with their achievements.
- The results and hard work spawn new willpower and ambition.
- The fruits give rise to gratitude and appreciation.

When, Why, What & How to Cleanse, for Everyone

This info is not a cleanse; it is, hopefully, just the info you need to figure out how to build the perfect cleanse PROGRAM for you. Note the word "program" refers to the fact that, ideally, cleansing is a process to improve upon year by year.

Once you read the info presented here and are ready to start a cleanse, go to the appropriate season and apply the guidelines learned right here in this section for your specific in-season cleanse.

<u>When</u>

No matter what is going on in my life, I have always felt my best when I stay in tune with nature and follow the laws of each season, such as Chinese medicine and other ancient cultures have learned and taught for thousands of years.

This means that I cleanse once per season (spring, summer, fall and winter) and that cleansing to me is not just nutrition but also about the mental, emotional and spiritual properties that align with each season. You will learn all of these properties as you read each seasonal cleanse.

Because one of my favorite benefits of cleansing is the discipline it gives me, I also like to do 1-3 day cleanses each month so that my discipline doesn't spiral out of control. These can be as simple as no meat or coffee for a day, fruits and veggies only for a day, or maybe a juice fast on a Sunday or anything else I may feel at that time.

Often times our discipline, or lack thereof, is most noticeable in what and how we eat, so I like to make sure that my eating does not get out of control and start affecting my discipline in other avenues of life, such as business, sleep patterns or spiritual practices.

It is astonishing how much one day of mindful eating can boost one's discipline and confidence in EVERYTHING else they do. Not to mention help the liver and other organs detoxify some of the poisons they have been ingesting on a daily basis.

Summary

- One major cleanse (1-3 weeks) each season (4)
- One minor cleanse (1-3 days) each month (12)

Why

The consequences of accumulating toxins in the body are chronic and degenerative diseases, immune system disorders, neurological disorders, digestive disorders, hormonal imbalances, cardio-vascular diseases, cancers, obesity, and more.

Cleansing is more important than ever

Nowadays we are exposed to more environmental toxins and pollutants than ever before in history and the need to detoxify on a regular basis has become essential for optimal health.

While there are many detoxification programs to choose from, it is important to choose a plan that one can actually follow and that respects the state of health one's body is in.

One of the worst things to do is start an intense cleanse if 1) the person has never done one before and 2) the body is relatively unhealthy and has a lot of toxins to release.

The following list is what we have proven time after time for centuries to be the bi-products of cleansing.

CLEANSES ARE ESSENTIAL FOR HEALTH because they...

- Nurture the digestive system. About 80% of our immune system and, therefore, ability to fight disease and illness resides in our gut
- Reduce the storage of toxins

- Provide the nutrients that support the detox pathways enhancing elimination of toxins
- Provide nutrients that help repair, renew and nourish the body
- Enhance discipline
- Promote getting in touch with nature and creating a healthy bio-rhythm
- Boost immunity by preventing an overloaded system and cleansing the blood
- Prevent chronic disease
- Reduce allergies
- Improve quality of life
- Encourage the loss of excess weight
- Improve the look and feel of skin
- Increase energy levels
- Reduce inflammation
- Balance hormones
- Increase the body's ability to cope with stress
- Give your physical body a vacation and promote better cellular communication and ability to fight disease
- Stop or slow premature aging by reducing oxidative stress (one of the biggest factors in premature aging) and free radical damage

Summary
- Cleansing prevents the accumulation of toxins, illness and disease.
- Cleanses promote well being, increased energy and optimum health.

What

Let's keep this simple, because as anyone who Googles™ "cleansing" knows (all 44,000,000 of them), this subject can become over complexified (yes, that is a word =). Usually, it seems that those who are selling something to help people cleanse are giving the most complicated explanations on the subject, and, of course, claiming that their products or treatment will cleanse people of whatever the toxic disease is.

While all of their claims may be true, the bigger question is this; are they really necessary? Are the products and various things they recommend actually needed to detox the specific parts of the body?

My hope is to make it clear that, unless one has a serious disease that has progressed to the point where intervention is necessary, most often one can encourage their body to adequately cleanse itself with very simple techniques.

After all, that is what it is created to do! It is our lifestyle and environment that hinder the natural process of detoxification. Once we get out of our own way, the body will take over and cleanse itself without much help at all.

What a wonderful machine we live in, right? Wouldn't it be nice if our car would change its own oil and filters if we just drove it right and let it rest 6-8 hours every night!?

The good news is that the body inherently gathers up and removes toxins from its cells and blood throughout the entire body every second of every day. The liver breaks them down and the kidneys, skin, colon, lungs, and mucus linings in the nose and ears get rid of them.

In other words, every time we've had bad breath, a coughing or sneezing attack, random stinkiness or sweating, or many other bodily "undesirables," we were probably just detoxing!

Okay, back to the *what*.

Detoxification refers to the process of eliminating toxins from the body. There are two major types of toxins the body accumulates over time:

Environmental Toxins: Also called exogenous (made outside of the body) toxins, include all the chemicals, pesticides, pollutants, herbicides, medications, carbon monoxides, and many, many, and, unfortunately, many more that we're exposed to through air, water, and food.

Metabolic Toxins: Also called endogenous (made inside the body) toxins, are produced by the cells as part of their natural metabolic processes or unnatural processes such as incompletely digested food microorganisms.

** It is normal for the cells to contain some toxins at all times.**

Toxins are only dangerous to one's health when allowed to accumulate so much so that they interfere with cellular function - which is called **toxicosis**.

My approach to cleansing is simple. I want to encourage my body to eliminate the two major types of toxins that accumulate on a daily basis. And since stress is a large factor, I include ways to rejuvenate the mental, emotional and spiritual aspects of life, as well as nutrition strategies.

I do not recommend or sell certain products, although I do use some natural herbs, teas, probiotics and some other natural-based aids to help the process.

I also do not promote any sort of "liver" cleanse, "colon" cleanse, or any other type of cleanse aimed at treating a certain organ. I will, however, give tips on what kind of herbs help specific organs function better based on research and science.

Can you see the difference? We are including the whole body here and not trying to fix anything in particular; simply encouraging the body to do what it's already doing, which is continually healing itself no matter how hard we try to screw it up.

Summary

- The goal of cleansing is to promote the body's natural ability to eliminate the two major types of toxins; environmental and metabolic.
- The philosophy here follows more of a total body approach than a specific organ or disease cleanse.

How

It can take months, years, even decades for toxins to build up enough to cause chronic disease and symptoms. For this reason, it is unrealistic to expect one cleanse to solve all of one's problems or even make a noticeable shift in overall health.

This is where cleansing with the seasons makes perfect sense as a lifestyle plan and something to build upon for as long as one is eating and breathing.

As mentioned before in the "What" section, the body is cleansing itself on a daily basis and does not require much in the way of specific regimens to experience a good amount of cleansing.

So if the seasonal approach below is too much for you to start with, try these *3 basic fundamentals* that facilitate the body's natural ability to cleanse itself.

1. Get as much physical, mental, and emotional rest as possible, and use fresh air, silence and sunshine to nurture spiritual energy.
2. Hydrate with water-rich foods (mostly fruits and vegetables) and liquids.
3. Minimize exposure to exogenous and endogenous toxins.

To cleanse with the seasons, keep reading.

Step 1
You want to make sure that you give yourself permission to set aside as much time as your life allows and to put in enough effort and intention to achieve a feeling of renewal. Cleansing halfway or in a rush is not going to give you that deep cleanse you are probably looking for, although it is at least a start.

Step 2
As mentioned in the "When" section, the most important part of cleansing/healing for me and many others who follow ancient medicine is to connect with and get into the rhythm of *nature* by cleansing with each season.

Before starting a cleanse, it is wise to prepare the body for it so there is not an abrupt change in your inner ecology, just like nature prepares the earth by having a transition period in between each season.

Most of us are unaware of this transition, but with some keen observation, one can notice that there is a great amount of energy taking place right before each season really gets going into its full force. Chinese medicine relates this transition period to the Earth element and energy.

For instance, in nature, Earth energy looks like the last winter storm that clears the air and waters the soil right before spring starts, or a fire at the end of summer to cleanse the soil for autumn. It is a very nurturing and supportive energy.

Please go to the *Earth Transition Cleanse* to read more about it and learn how to start each cleanse off on the right foot and prepare the body to deeply take in and reap all the benefits from whatever cleanse you choose to do.

Step 3

Before starting a cleanse, it is essential to know where your health is at so you know exactly what you are getting into. For example, if you have never cleansed before, you probably should not start with an intermediate or advanced cleanse, unless, of course, you are prepared to suffer and have a lot of wherewithal to survive the process!

The most common mistake I see with cleansing is that people get gung ho about detoxing and choose an aggressive cleanse to start with. There is nothing really wrong with that; however, it is a very intense way to do it and is usually the exact opposite thing that most people need, which is more intensity in their life.

That said, my first cleanse was very intense, and I am lucky to still have a yearning to do more because of what I went through. I had intense headaches for three days, among other discomforts, was pissed off and irritated more people in that time than I probably have in the many years since.

So, my advice is always the same, ease into cleansing and take an approach about it that allows you to improve upon your successes each time. The beauty of cleansing is that the body actually learns to recognize the patterns of it and becomes more efficient each time it goes through the process, like a cleansing memory.

Once the body has some experience with cleansing, all you need is the intention to cleanse, and then the body automatically starts its detoxification processes (before the cleanse actually starts) just like it increases its saliva when the brain thinks about food.

Below are some guidelines I have learned that are great for helping people decide where to start and how much they can handle. Everyone is in different places with their health, discipline and time/effort allowances relating to work, life, etc.

Do not over commit, take it easy, and choose components that you feel comfortable with and can achieve without much difficulty the first time.

This is a general list that will be expanded upon with each seasonal cleanse.
1-3 weeks is a good amount of time to allow for deep cleansing.

The goals are to choose components that 1) you need to work on and 2) can hopefully, be maintained somewhat post-cleansing, and thus use them as a new-found health tool to build upon.

This method of "chipping away" at one's weaknesses will smoothly transition a person from beginner to wherever they wish to end up.

Figure out where to start right here.

Beginner	Intermediate	Master
• Choose at least 3 components from EACH list	• Choose at least 10 components from EACH list	• Do ALL components from each list.

TO DO LIST   (choose 3/10/or all)

- Sleep pattern; example, 10:30pm-6:30am
- Organic, free-range foods
- Grass fed, no-hormone beef
- Follow the **80/20 rules***
- 10 min stretching daily
- 10 min silence/meditation daily
- 20 min walking daily (ideally outside with fresh air)
- 10 min plugging into nature (observe in silence any way you wish)
- Proper **food combining***
- Proper **blood type foods***
- Follow **cooking & eating rules***
- Eat *simple meals*, i.e. only 2-3 types of food each meal, including types of veggies
- Increase your **antioxidants***
- Eat as **alkaline*** as possible
- Eat fresh, seasonal fruits and veggies throughout the day

See Appendix

ELIMINATION LIST (choose 3/10/or all)

- Complaining
- The **No-No List***
- Negative self talk
- **Allergy foods***
- T.V. and news
- All fats but coconut oil and olive oil
- Added salt
- Overcooked foods
- Gluten and wheat
- **Refined sugar***
- Processed foods
- Meat (all types)
- Nuts and seeds
- Processed dairy (anything not raw)
- Overeating
- Foods on your blood type **"avoid" list***
- Unhealthy cleaning or beauty products
- Violence, hate, anger, etc. (movies, books, people, music, etc.)

See Appendix

THE MUST FOLLOW LIST *(yes, all of them)*

Avoid
- Alcohol
- Coffee
- Soda
- Microwaved or canned food
- Super intense physical activity
- Smoking and recreational drugs
- Overworking, over-committing, etc.

Do
- *Earth Transition Cleanse*
- Use breathing to release stress and tension throughout the day.
- Drink half your body weight in ounces of water; 100lb person should drink 50 ounces of water per day.
- Get as much physical, mental, and emotional rest as possible, and use fresh air, silence and sunshine whenever available to nurture your spiritual energy.

X-FACTORS

1) AVOID VARIOUS TOXINS - One could do everything right in their cleanse and still not get a good detox if they miss these X-factors.

Besides good nutrition, mental and emotional practices, one also must avoid ingesting various toxic chemicals or putting them on their skin, because the body can absorb many toxic chemicals through the skin. From the skin they will seep into the blood stream and lymphatic system, eventually accumulating wherever they are attracted to.

Below are only a few areas to focus on and are essential for health on a daily basis, whether one is cleansing or not.

- Air, food and water
- Health products (toiletries, cosmetics, deodorants, etc.)
- Cleaning supplies
- Smoking and drug addictions (including over-the-counter drugs)
- Environmental: fumes, smoke, chemicals, STRESS, etc.

2) RELEASE STORED TOXINS - The goal here is to add some methods that encourage the body to release any harmful chemicals that are presently stored in the body. The cleanses presented for each season also promote the release of toxins, but these are a few things to do in general to facilitate the process even more.

- Drink lots of water (promotes release through urine, which is the preferred method of releasing toxins)
- Massages, acupuncture, etc. (promotes blood flow and stimulates areas to release stored tension and toxins)
- Clay baths (helps release excess metals)
- Neti pot (releases bacteria build up in nasal cavities)
- Sweat, i.e. exercise, walk, steam room, etc.
- Fasting. There are many ways to fast, which give the body a rest from digesting and lets it focus on detoxing; this is an advanced method and takes experience or professional guidance.

3) Rest - Simple, obvious, yet the most often overlooked factor, is rest. Give the body the rest it needs so it can devote its resources to cleansing and detoxifying mechanisms.

Summary

Step 1
Make sure your life (job, family, time, etc.) can support your cleanse and that you are mentally ready and have set intentions.

Step 2
Cleanse with each season and start by preparing the body for your "real" cleanse by doing a transition cleanse. The *Earth Transition Cleanse* is what I recommend.

Step 3
Decide which level of cleanser you are, beginner, intermediate, or master, and choose your components accordingly.

WARNING

There is something known as the "Cleansing Reaction" that you should know about...

When the body starts its process of eliminating toxins, there can be "un-fun" symptoms during this time. And as a rule, the more toxins and gunk one has stored in their tissues, the more uncomfortable this process is going to be, which is why I recommend cleansing at the appropriate level; i.e., beginner, intermediate or advanced.

This is also why one should have an intention and clear focus before doing a cleanse; otherwise it is easy to be derailed and turned off from cleansing forever.

There are numerous ways to release toxins; here are just a few along with their symptoms. As long as one follows a proper cleanse, these are all good things, just not very fun to go through.

Natural Ways the Body Releases Toxins	What We May Feel or Notice
The Skin	Rashes, reddish bumps, etc.
Mucous	Runny nose, phlegm, coughing, etc.
Urine	Darker color, smelly, frequent need to urinate, etc.

Gases	Bad breath or gas
Blood & Lymph (they are transported temporarily here before being released)	Headaches, lethargy, frustration, irritability, sweating, filmy tongue, and more
Experiencing	Stored memories, traumas, drugs, etc. can be released into the body and re-create their original feelings associated with that experience; i.e., drug users can feel "high" when detoxing from their drugs because the drugs are released into the blood on their way out of the body

Spring Cleanse

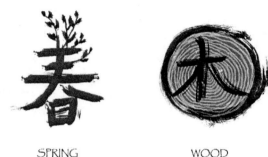

SPRING   WOOD

Spring is a time for leaving the stillness of winter and promoting new life, creativity, dreams, goal setting, planning, cleansing, assertiveness and the many other attributes associated with the Wood element and spring energy you will learn in this cleanse.

If you are experienced at cleansing, this is often the best time to do your biggest cleanse of the year, you know, "spring cleaning."

"An optimist is the human personification of spring." ~ Susan J. Bissonette

In Chinese medicine, everyone falls into a dominant element, (Fire, Earth, Metal, Water or Wood). Although we always have all 5 elements running through us, we tend to have one that is strongest in our personalities, strengths, weaknesses, etc. You can get an idea of where your strongest element is here...
http://lotusinstitute.com/5ElementsQuiz.html

Healing may not be so much about getting better as about letting go of everything that isn't you—all of the expectations, all of the beliefs—and becoming who you are. Not a better you, but a realer you. ~ Rachael Naomi Remen, M.D., The Human Patient (Anchor Books, 1980)

This Spring cleanse includes all dimensions of health, not just nutrition, and remember that by practicing the mental, emotional and spiritual aspects of this cleanse, you will automatically be healing the organs related to Spring, which are the liver and gall bladder.

The emotions and attitudes you will be focusing on here are exactly what feed or starve the exact organs related to spring; i.e., anger and poor decision making deplete the liver and gall bladder, while assertiveness and forgiveness build them up.

Guidelines

- Start with the **Earth Transition Cleanse**.
- While the focus is a total body cleanse, the organs related to spring are the liver and gall bladder, so many of the intentions in the MESP Focus are set around these two organs, which encourages the rest of the body to follow in the detoxification process of Spring.
- This is a **21-day cleanse**. If you are a beginner, then you can cut each week in half and progress each year from there.

Week # 1

- Select your level, *beginner/ intermediate/master; see "Cleanse Options List" in the Appendix and* follow the guidelines from the ***To Do List*** and the ***Elimination List*** (Choose 3, 10 or all from each list)
- Follow the guidelines in the Spring MESP Focus
- Eat lots of fresh, seasonal fruits and vegetables (local is best)

Week # 2

- Same as week 1
- 1-7 day juice fast*
- Move up to the next level; i.e., if you are a beginner, move up to intermediate this week*
- Take a vacation/retreat this week to focus solely on the cleanse*
- Take a psyllium husk mixture** in water every morning and night on an empty stomach (1T in 8 ounces water)*
- Drink the master cleanse** mixture 1-2x per day*

*Optional
**See Appendix for more info

Week # 3

- Same as week # 1, but ease back into it if you did more intense cleansing in week # 2

Mental, Emotional, Spiritual and Physical (MESP) Focus

Just as the body cannot exist without blood, so the soul needs the matchless and pure strength of faith. ~Mahatma Gandhi

MENTAL

1. Set goals for the entire year and make plans to achieve them (any part of life).
2. Balance your responsibilities; let go of any that are too much or not yours, and only take on those that you can handle.

EMOTIONAL

1. Observe the ebbs and flows of your spring energy;

    - too much energy = anger/frustration
    - too little energy = unassertive/passive
    - just right = **assertive**

2. Forgive anything or anyone necessary to move on with your cleanse or life in general. This includes forgiving yourself.

3. Repeat the following mantras once in the morning and once in the evening.

   - I am Confident
   - I am Assertive
   - I am Bold
   - I am Ambitious
   - I am Competitive
   - I am Powerful
   - I am Direct
   - I am Committed
   - I am Decisive

SPIRITUAL

1. The Pioneer is the archetype for spring (Wood element), so focus on blazing your own path with your goals.
2. Write down what your big dreams are (own a house, travel, have children, teach, etc.) and be very descriptive.
3. Focus on strengthening or finding your purpose.
4. Focus on "being" rather than winning.
5. "Be aware the bareness of a busy life." ~ Socrates
6. Embrace asking others for help.

7. This is a time for dreaming, not rigidity. Let your mind go and think about all the things you used to want and maybe forgot about. No intentions, simply dreaming.

PHYSICAL

1. Drink detox teas in the morning and evening made from one or more of the following herbs (many stores already have teas like this for liver detoxing and cleansing); milk thistle, turmeric, artichoke extract, rosemary, dandelion, yellow dock, gentian, green tea, barberry.
2. Clean out the garage, closet, car, desk, etc.
3. Focus on being grounded like a tree, flexible yet strong. This is best done by simply observing a tree in the winds of spring and standing in a strong position such as horse stance (see next page).

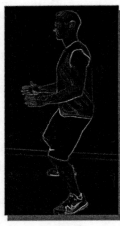

Horse Stance

Assume a strong stance as in the picture to the left. Practice feeling 1) strongly grounded, 2) energy between your hands, as if hugging a tree and feeling its power from the ground up, and 3) nature by looking or being outside during this stance.

Start the morning with this stance to assure a grounded feeling throughout the rest of day. Stay here for 5-30 minutes!

Summer Cleanse

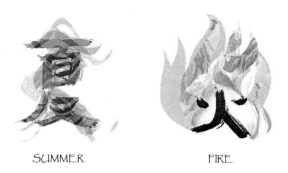

SUMMER   FIRE

Metaphorically, Summer is a time for blossoming and flourishing, focusing and following through, joy and the anticipation of success. Imagine planting seeds (goals) in spring, now you must water (which means focusing on goals and plans) and weed (remove or overcome obstacles) in order for your crop (goal) to come to fruition (in autumn).

    This cleanse is all about staying focused on your goals, following through with what you've started, and having JOY and enthusiasm while doing it. The farmer or the chef will not create a great harvest or meal if their efforts are joyless.

The work it takes to obtain your goals should stem from the joy that the goals will bring; very simple, but often forgotten. The reason gramma's meals taste so yummy is because she cooks with love and joy.

Your goals and hard work are no different. The pursuit of goals with methodical and lifeless energy will bring about the "gifts" of emptiness. The pursuit of goals with joy and anticipation of success will bring a deep contentment with your efforts and encourage the pursuit of similar things naturally.

The Summer cleanse is not a big cleanse compared to that of spring, because it is a continuation of what you have already started instead of a completely new journey.

Love the moment. Flowers grow out of dark moments. Therefore, each moment is vital. It affects the whole. Life is a succession of such moments and to live each, is to succeed.
~ Corina Kent

Just like the spring cleanse, the mental, emotional, spiritual and physical aspects of Summer will be practiced here to facilitate the powers needed to feel joy, focus and follow through with your intentions.

"The season of failure is the best time for sowing the seeds of success." ~ Paramahansa Yogananda

This Summer cleanse includes all dimensions of health, not just nutrition, and remember that by practicing the mental, emotional and spiritual aspects of this cleanse, you will automatically be healing the organs* related to Summer, the heart and small intestine.

The emotions and attitudes you will be focusing on here are exactly what feed or starve the exact organs related to Summer; i.e., sadness starves the heart while joy and happiness feed it.

*Please note that there are two other non-Western organs included in Summer, or the Fire element. They are circulation sex and triple warmer. For simplicity's sake, they will be left out of this cleanse, although they will be indirectly cleansed from the steps below.

Guidelines

- Start with the **Earth Transition Cleanse**.

- While the focus is a total body cleanse, the organs related to Summer are the heart and small intestine, so many of the intentions in the MESP Focus are set around these two organs, which encourages the rest of the body to follow in the detoxification process of summer.
- This is a **10-21 day cleanse**, depending on your level, commitment and needs.
- The large variation in time for this cleanse depends on where you are at with your health and goals.
- This cleanse can be used as a quick health enhancer for 10 days to boost discipline and the immune system.
- The main week contains at least 3 days of nutritional cleansing and 7 days of mental, emotional, spiritual and physical cleansing related to Summer.

Week # 1

- Week 1 is an optional "easing into the cleanse" period (1-7 days)
- Select your level, *beginner/intermediate/master; see "Cleanse Options List" in the Appendix and* follow the guidelines from the ***To Do List*** and the

Elimination List (Choose 3, 10 or all from each list)
- Follow guidelines in MESP Focus for summer

Week # 2

- Mandatory (7 days)
- Follow the guidelines from the ***To Do List*** and the ***Elimination List*** (Choose 3, 10 or all)~ ***at least 3 days***
- Follow MESP Focus for the summer *(7 days)*
- 1-3 day juice fast*
- Move up to the next level; i.e., if you are beginner, move up to intermediate this week*
- Take a vacation/retreat this week to focus solely on the cleanse*
- Take a psyllium husk mixture** in water every morning and night on an empty stomach (1T in 8 ounces water)~ ***at least 3 days****
- Drink the master cleanse mixture** 1-2x per day*

    *Optional
    ** See Appendix for more info

Week # 3

- Mandatory (3-7 days)

- Follow the guidelines from the ***To Do List*** and the ***Elimination List*** (Choose 3, 10 or all)~ ***at least 3 days***
- Ease back into regular lifestyle and eating habits

Mental, Emotional, Spiritual and Physical (MESP) Focus

We act as though comfort and luxury were the chief requirements of life, when all that we need to make us really happy is something to be enthusiastic about. ~Charles Kingsley

MENTAL

1. Make a list of things that you need to follow through with and create an action plan to finish them. Most importantly, *enjoy* finishing them by anticipating their success.

For each goal you are following through with, perform a 5 minute daily visualization on what it will feel and look like when you have successfully completed it. Be very specific and go into as much detail as imaginable.

This may seem silly, but it is one of the most proven and powerful ways to attract success, or anything else, for that matter. If you ask people who are very successful, no matter what it is, they often visualize their actions and results before they ever happen.

2. Make a list of things that you enjoy and don't enjoy doing. Then, figure out how to 1) spend more time doing the things you enjoy, and 2) better enjoy the things you don't enjoy.

EMOTIONAL

1. Observe the ebbs and flows of your Summer energy;
- too much energy = hysteria/over-excitement/anxious
- too little energy = gloomy/melancholy/confused/selfish/panicky
- just right = j**oy**

2. Focus on positivity and simply observing any negative thoughts, while letting go of these negative thoughts through your breath.

3. Repeat the following mantras once in the morning and once in the evening.
- I am happy and joyful
- I am focused on my goals
- I am enjoying my journey

- I follow through with what I start
- I am anticipating success
- I am flourishing
- I am tender and empathetic
- I am a great communicator
- I am optimistic
- I am aware
- I am enthusiastic and devoted

SPIRITUAL

1. The Wizard is the archetype of Fire/Summer, so focus on being the eye of the storm and remaining calm when surrounded by chaos. This is done with breathing and observing instead of reacting or judging.
2. Take 5-10 minutes of daily silence while focusing solely on what brings you joy and helps you flourish. Practice this silence with a smile on your face as if you were actually experiencing the events.

PHYSICAL

1. Do physical activities that you really enjoy. Going for walks with loved ones, dancing, riding a bike and whatever else gets you moving

outside in the fresh air. Keep intensity to moderate levels so the body can heal itself.

2. Get some sun, daily.

3. For your heart, encourage healing by refraining from intense activity and focusing on keeping your heart rate at its resting rate as much as possible

Autumn Cleanse

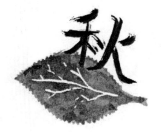

AUTUMN

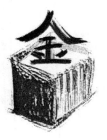

METAL

The second biggest cleanse of the year is Autumn, behind spring. It is a time for letting go and reaping what you sow. Realizing your progress and all of your accomplishments is essential for enjoying the journey through Autumn and its associated element, Metal.

"Autumn is a second spring when every leaf is a flower." ~ Albert Camus

It is in Autumn that nature and the farmer are working their magic and harvesting huge crops which started out as small seedlings. This is where one should receive gifts for all of their hard work. Finishing tasks and completing goals are the main energies at work.

Compassion is the energy that guides you through the completion of goals to make sure rewards are at their potential. Nothing is worse than working hard all the way until the end and then slowing down at the finish line. The best results are had when you charge *through* the finish line.

For man, autumn is a time of harvest, of gathering together. For nature, it is a time of sowing, of scattering abroad. ~ Edwin Way Teale

This Autumn cleanse includes all dimensions of health, not just nutrition, and remember that, by practicing the mental, emotional and spiritual aspects of this cleanse, you will automatically be healing the organs related to Autumn, which are the lungs and large intestine.

The emotions and attitudes you will be focusing on here are exactly what feed or starve the exact organs related to Autumn; i.e., receiving and completing things encourages the function of the lungs and large intestine while grief and sadness disrupt them.

Guidelines

- Start with the **Earth Transition Cleanse**.
- While the focus is a total body cleanse, the organs related to autumn are the lungs and large intestine, so many of the intentions in the MESP Focus are set around these two organs, which encourages the rest of the body to follow in the detoxification process of autumn.
- This is a **21-day cleanse**. If you are a beginner, then you can cut each week in half and progress each year from there.

Week # 1

- Select your level, *beginner/intermediate/master; see "Cleanse Options List" in the Appendix and* follow the guidelines from the ***To Do List*** and the ***Elimination List*** (Choose 3, 10 or all from each list)
- Follow guidelines in Autumn MESP Focus
- Eat warmer foods like fresh soups and stews instead of salads to get your body used to the cooler weather and ready for winter

Week # 2

- Same as week 1

- 1-7 day juice fast*
- Move up to the next level; i.e., if you are a beginner, move up to intermediate this week*
- Take a vacation/retreat this week to focus solely on the cleanse*
- Take a psyllium husk mixture** in water every morning and night on an empty stomach (1T in 8 ounces water)*
- Drink the master cleanse mixture** 1-2x per day*

*Optional
**See Appendix for more details

Week # 3

- Same as week # 1, but ease back into it if you did more intense cleansing in week # 2

Mental, Emotional, Spiritual and Physical (MESP) Focus

"How beautifully things grow old. How full of light and color are their last days." ~ John Burroughs

MENTAL

1. Finish what you start. Everything is about letting go and completing in autumn. Create habits of completing tasks without handing off the responsibility whenever applicable.
2. Practice accepting and receiving things such as gifts and compliments. This is the time to cash in on all the hard work put into spring and summer.

EMOTIONAL

1. Observe the ebbs and flows of your Autumn energy;

- too much energy = grief, sadness and regret
- too little energy = apathy and indifference
- just right = **compassion**

2. Let go of any things, ideas or people holding you back. Use relaxed breathing (lungs are related to Autumn) to let go of energies not supporting you, just like the trees letting go of their leaves.

3. Repeat the following mantras once in the morning and once in the evening.

- I am methodical and discerning
- I accept and receive all the good that comes my way
- I am calm and disciplined
- I am precise
- I am reserved
- I let go of things that do not support me
- I complete what I start
- I am compassionate

SPIRITUAL

1. Realize how much you have grown while on your journey since spring.
2. The Alchemist is the archetype of Autumn (the metal element), so focus on turning seeds into fruits and sins into virtues.
3. Absorb yourself in 5-10 minutes of daily silence on purity and honesty.

PHYSICAL

1. Use a neti pot and breathe in hot steam filled with a few drops of eucalyptus oil or herbs to cleanse the lungs and sinuses of allergies and congestions that have accumulated throughout

the year, especially when the leaves start falling and rotting.

2. Clean out your garage, closet, car, desk, etc., and throw out or sell (let go) any unnecessary items.

3. Nurture your lungs with lots of fresh, clean air to breathe while you take daily walks outside.

4. Use natural herbal teas to keep the body warm. Some stores already have great general detoxification teas available.

Winter Cleanse

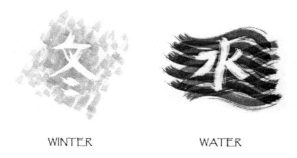

WINTER   WATER

The Winter cleanse is similar to the summer cleanse; both are aimed at continuing the momentum of the previous season rather than a total makeover of the body's systems. Winter is a time for rest and reflection so that learning and future cycles are built from realizing our mistakes and successes.

"Let us love winter, for it is the spring of genius." ~ Pietro Aretino

It is in Winter that nature and the farmer are laying low and resting from a busy year. This is where energy, wisdom and reserves are built up for another busy year to come when spring arrives.

Cautiousness is a dominant force during this time because it is all too easy to waste energy and completely miss the lessons from the whole year. Winter is a great teacher for conserving energy and realizing the big picture of life's cycles.

Continuing to live life as intensely as usual in the wintertime is like trying to accomplish things at night instead of sleeping.

"The color of springtime is in the flowers, the color of winter is in the imagination." ~ *Terri Guillemets*

This Winter cleanse includes all dimensions of health, not just nutrition, and remember that by practicing the mental, emotional and spiritual aspects of this cleanse, you will automatically be healing the organs related to winter, which are the kidneys and bladder.

The emotions and attitudes you will be focusing on here are exactly what feed or starve the exact organs related to Winter; i.e., resting and contemplating things encourages the function of the kidney and bladder while fear and terror disrupt them.

Guidelines

- Start with the **Earth Transition Cleanse**.
- While the focus is a total body cleanse, the organs related to Winter are the kidney and the bladder, so many of the intentions in the MESP Focus are set around these two organs, which encourages the rest of the body to follow in the detoxification process of winter.
- This is a **<u>10-21 day cleanse</u>**, depending on your level, commitment and needs.
- The large variation in time for this cleanse depends on where you are at with your health and goals.
- This cleanse can be used as a quick health enhancer for 10 days to boost discipline and the immune system.
- The main week contains at least 3 days of nutritional cleansing and 7 days of mental, emotional, spiritual and physical cleansing related to winter.

<u>Week # 1</u>

- Week 1 is an optional "easing into the cleanse" period (1-7 days)
- Select your level, *beginner/ intermediate/master; see "Cleanse Options*

List" in the Appendix and follow the guidelines from the *To Do List* and the ***Elimination List*** (Choose 3, 10 or all from each list)
- Follow guidelines in MESP Focus for winter

Week # 2

- Mandatory (7 days)
- Follow the guidelines from the ***To Do List*** and the ***Elimination List*** (Choose 3, 10 or all)~ *at least 3 days*
- Follow MESP Focus for the winter (7 days)
- 1-3 day juice fast*
- Move up to the next level; i.e., if you are beginner, move up to intermediate this week*
- Take a vacation/retreat this week to focus solely on the cleanse*
- Take a psyllium husk mixture** in water every morning and night on an empty stomach (1T in 8 ounces water) ~ *at least 3 days**
- Drink the <u>master cleanse</u> mixture** 1-2x per day*

*Optional
**See Appendix for more details

Week # 3

- Mandatory (3-7 days)
- Follow the guidelines from the ***To Do List*** and the ***Elimination List*** (Choose 3, 10 or all)~ ***at least 3 days***
- Ease back into regular lifestyle and eating habits.

Mental, Emotional, Spiritual and Physical (MESP) Focus

"Winter must be cold for those with no warm memories." ~From the movie "An Affair to Remember"

MENTAL

1. This is a time to look back on your accomplishments, evaluate and appreciate them. Learn from your journey so that next year you will be that much better and more in tune with nature.
2. Practice willpower, you will need it if you are someone who persistently needs to be doing things. This is a time for rest and reflection, not

constant motion. Less is more during wintertime.

3. Once reflection and evaluation of the year have finished, this down time is well spent on playing with ambitious thoughts for the following year.

A lot of time is needed for reflection and evaluation, so resist the urge to rush through the energy of this season, because without the proper rest and reflection, the next year will be malnourished.

EMOTIONAL

1. Observe the ebbs and flows of your winter energy;

- too much energy = terror and fear
- too little energy = careless and reckless
- just right = **cautious**

2. Let go of any things, ideas or people holding you back. Use relaxed breathing (lungs related to autumn) to let go of energies not supporting you, just like the trees letting go of their leaves.

3. Repeat the following mantras once in the morning and once in the evening.

- I am introspective right now
- I am modest
- I am watchful
- I am careful
- I am thrifty and sensible
- I am clear
- I am open and honest
- I am objective
- I am grateful
- I am particular

SPIRITUAL

1. The archetype of Winter (the Water element) is the Philosopher, so focus on Self contemplation and tapping into the infinite wisdom of the universe.
2. Rest, reflect, store and conserve.
3. Absorb yourself in 5-10 minutes of daily reflection about how far your Self has come this year.

PHYSICAL

1. REST. Lower the intensity wherever possible.
2. Keep your body healthy with exercise and stretching, but keep them simple and moderate.

3. Use natural herbal teas to keep the body warm. Some stores already have great general detoxification teas available.

Earth Cleanse

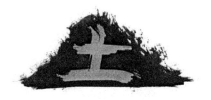

EARTH

Earth's energy is the focus used at the beginning of each seasonal cleanse because it is thought to be the transition phase between each season, rather than its own season. It is the energy that nurtures and supports all other seasons.

This is a time in nature where the most energy often occurs, as transitions require a complete shift in the direction of energy and growth. For this reason, it is included as a pre-cleanse in order to get the body prepared mentally, emotionally, spiritually and physically.

Think of Earth energy as the curving angle that connects two perpendicular roads smoothly like an on or off-ramp, thus allowing a nice transition without much slowing down at all. Compare this to an abrupt 90 degree change of direction that usually requires a stop sign.

In nature, Earth energy looks like the last winter storm that clears the air and waters the wood (which is the spring element), or a fire at the end of summer to cleanse the soil.

The Earth Transition Cleanse has 3 components to follow every day, for 3-7 days

These 3-7 days are prior to any and all of the seasonal cleanses. Each of the following components are based on the qualities, smells, colors, etc. that are associated with the Earth element.

1. Mantras - Repeat the following while thinking of the color yellow and *feeling* what each word means. Repeat once in the morning and once in the evening.

- I am loving
- I am peaceful
- I have faith
- I am gentle

- I am patient
- I have integrity
- I am kind
- I am generous
- I am loyal
- I am tolerant
- I am sympathetic
- I am nurturing and supportive
- I am relaxed
- I am sociable
- I am considerate
- I am poised
- I am attentive
- I am here to serve

2. ***Intention*** – Envision what health is to YOU. What it feels like. What it looks like. How it would change your life. Who you would hang out with, and who you wouldn't. What you look like when you're healthy, etc. Do this in the following four ways.

1. Draw it
2. Sing/speak it
3. Envision it
4. Dance it

Trust me, singing and dancing are not my thing either, but it is one of the few and most efficient ways to tap into and influence of the sub and unconscious minds. If you can't access those parts of your mind, you are acting one-dimensional, at best.

These four distinct ways are essential for combining all of your senses together to give you a complete picture of health to resonate with and, therefore, attract your body to in a very, very powerful way (try it while driving in your car =)

3. *Observation* – Observe your body during this time if it ebbs and flows through anxiety and depression, and when you are in harmony.

Use the mantras to restore your harmony when you notice yourself slipping into too much Earth energy (anxiety) or not enough Earth energy (depression).

Off-Season Nutrition

So what does one do when they are not cleansing with the seasons? Well, that depends on whether a person is a) cleansing because they want to consistently improve how they eat and feel or b) simply cleansing away their terrible eating habits only to return to those same habits soon after.

If you are the "a" person, keep reading. If you are the "b" person, you're probably not even reading this!

Once someone finishes a cleanse, they should invariably pick up good habits that they did not previously have, or rarely practiced. That is *step one*; to keep as many good habits as possible from the cleanse and execute them as often as possible.

Step two is an extension of step one; to develop a program that utilizes as many tools from the cleanse as possible and lays out guidelines for what types of foods to eat and to stay away from.

Since the key to life is moderation and happiness, there should be cheat days or meals in this program, depending on one's health situation.

If someone is relatively healthy, then the program can be more lenient; but if someone is suffering from disease, then the program should be more strict and focused on healing the digestive system.

The beauty of cleansing is that a person often finds out which foods cause bloating, fatigue, congestion, headaches and even more symptoms of dis-ease. These "enlightenments" hopefully lead to the elimination of certain foods and the attraction to other foods that increase energy, stamina, mental clarity and the like.

After enough cleanses a person should be in total harmony with what their body likes and dislikes without even trying because they have trained themselves to eat in a way that naturally cleanses their systems.

In other words, the OFF-SEASON PROGRAM IS THIS:

- Follow as many tools as possible that you learned and enjoyed in the cleanse.
- Each time you cleanse, you will most likely add a tool or two to your off-season program.
- Eventually you will be constantly eating in a way that cleanses your body - how cool is that?!

APPENDIX

Cleanse Options List
Food Combining and Layering
Antioxidants
Allergy Foods
Cooking and Eating Rules
Primary Nutrition
Super Alkalizers
Inflammation Fighters
The No-No List
Refined vs. Natural Carbs
Master Cleanse Recipe
Psyllium Husk Mixture
Yin Yang Foods
Coconut Oil
80/20 Rules
Blood Type Foods

Cleanse Options List

Figure out where to start right here.

Beginner	Intermediate	Master
• Choose at least 3 components from EACH list	• Choose at least 10 components from EACH list	• Do ALL components from each list.

TO DO LIST (choose 3/10/or all)

- Sleep pattern; example, 10:30pm-6:30am
- Organic, free-range foods
- Grass fed, no-hormone beef
- Follow the **80/20 rules***
- 10 min stretching daily
- 10 min silence/meditation daily
- 20 min walking daily (ideally outside with fresh air)
- 10 min plugging into nature (observe in silence any way you wish)
- Proper **food combining***
- Proper **blood type foods***

- Follow **cooking & eating rules***
- Eat *simple meals*; i.e., only 2-3 types of food each meal, including types of veggies
- Increase your **antioxidants***
- Eat as **alkaline*** as possible
- Eat fresh, seasonal fruits and veggies throughout the day

See Appendix

ELIMINATION LIST (choose 3/10/or all)

- Complaining
- The **No-No List***
- Negative self talk
- **Allergy foods***
- T.V. and news
- All fats but coconut oil and olive oil
- Added salt
- Overcooked foods
- Gluten and wheat
- **Refined sugar***
- Processed foods
- Meat (all types)
- Nuts and seeds
- Processed dairy (anything not raw)
- Overeating
- Foods on your blood type **"avoid" list***

- Unhealthy cleaning or beauty products
- Violence, hate, anger, etc. (movies, books, people, music, etc.)

See Appendix

THE MUST FOLLOW LIST *(yes, all of them)*

Avoid
- Alcohol
- Coffee
- Soda
- Microwaved or canned food
- Super intense, physical activity
- Smoking and recreational drugs
- Overworking, over-committing, etc.

Do
- *Earth transition cleanse*
- Use breathing to release stress and tension throughout the day.
- Drink half your body weight in ounces of water; 100lb person should drink 50 ounces of water per day.
- Get as much physical, mental, and emotional rest as possible, and use fresh air, silence and sunshine to nurture your spiritual energy.

Food Combining and Layering

What is Food Combining?

Food combining is the art of giving your stomach the right foods at one meal so that it has the ideal combination of digestive juices needed to break down whatever is in the stomach.

Sugars, proteins and fats all need different digestive juices in order to be properly digested. If they are all mixed together, then each digestive concoction becomes diluted and unable to fully break down its specific food. This leads to improper assimilation, bloating and more.

What is Food Layering?

Food layering is the art of giving your stomach the right foods in the right order so that it has the ideal combination of digestive juices needed to break down whatever is in the stomach.

As food layering expert Dr. Stanley Bass[2] puts it;

Any quick digesting foods must wait till the slowest digesting foods leave the stomach before they can leave - a process which can take up to 6 or 8 hours. While waiting, the fruit, cooked and raw vegetables, and some of the starches undergo some decomposition and fermentation, producing gas, acid and even alcohol along with indigestion...

And...
... If there are 5 different types of food in the stomach at one meal, each eaten separately and in sequence, there will be 5 different kinds of digestion going on at the same time, each layer having different enzymes digesting each food, according to the needs of the food contained in that layer...But when say 5 different foods are eaten at a meal, where each mouthful or bite is taken of a different food, then the entire stomach is filled with the same mixture.

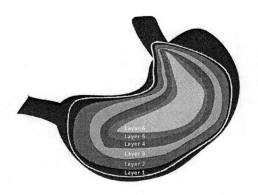

Image of ideal food layering; each food has its own digestive sack or layer and is able to fully break down its specific food without interference from antagonistic digestive juices. Layer 1 in this case was eaten first, followed by 2-6 sequentially.

So what's the difference between food combining and layering? With layering, one can basically eat whatever foods they want at a meal, as long as they are eaten in the proper order; i.e., the most watery foods first and proteins last. This tends to work very well, although not as well as when coupled with proper food combining guidelines.

Why Combine and Layer Food Properly?

Because most food cannot be assimilated in its natural state and needs to be converted into easily absorbable microparticles; our delivery mechanisms (how we eat, cook and store foods) are the secret to optimum health.

Correctly combining and layering foods is essential for **optimum digestion and assimilation**. Improper food combining, layering and poor nutrient absorption contribute to and can even be the main reasons people have bloating, indigestion, diarrhea, gas, upset stomach, arthritis, asthma, allergies, chronic fatigue, aches and pains, poor memory, disorganized thoughts and more.

Without proper digestion, nutrients in even the most wholesome of foods cannot be fully extracted and used by the body.

The goal is not to be a perfect food combiner, at least not at first. There are many things to learn and practice with this topic. So to make sure one gets the most out of it, look at it as a self-experiment when eating.

With a little practice and awareness, one will save their gut a lot of discomfort, get the most out of their food, lose weight if needed, and, most importantly, stop flooding the blood with waste bi-products from all the food that is spoiling in their stomach from being combined or layered incorrectly.

*Do not believe any of this info,
simply try it and judge for yourself.*

Basic Guidelines for Food Combining and Layering

1. Follow the food combining and layering rules whenever possible (see next pages and links). *Layering is most important and should be done even when following proper food combining rules.*
2. When ideal food combining can't be had, focus on layering the foods properly.
3. When neither can be followed, make sure indigestion, bloating and gas are acceptable for the following hours to come =)

Basic Rule of Food Layering:

1. Eat the most watery food first, followed by the second most watery, and so on.

Basic Rules of Proper Food Combining:

Here are 5 tools to start with. You can find more at the blog **http://tinyurl.com/7pyhub5** *which includes extensive charts on food combining. Remember, these are tools to improve digestion. See which of them make the biggest impact on your health and use them as often as possible.*

1. Do NOT eat <u>protein foods and carbohydrate foods at the same meals</u>. Protein foods require an acid medium for digestion while carbs/starches require the opposite. *Food layering modification*; eat the starches first, then the protein.

2. <u>Eat fruits alone</u> on an empty stomach and wait 20–30 min before eating again. *Food layering modification*; eat the fruit first, then the heavier foods.

3. Have <u>desserts and sugars by themselves</u> as its own meal, not right after a meal.

4. <u>No cold water or more than 4 ounces of liquids with meals</u>. One may consume 4 ounces of warm tea or water, kombucha or apple cider vinegar as

liquids to aid digestion. Otherwise no additional liquid fifteen minutes before or until 60 minutes after a meal.

5. Don't eat <u>high-fat foods and proteins at the same meal.</u> Keep the fats to a very small amount. Some foods, especially nuts, are over 50% fat and require hours to digest, which slows all other digestion.

Antioxidants

Please note there are many more foods, these just have the most per serving.

Berries (especially blueberries)
Green leafy veggies (especially kale)
Raw cacao
Sea veggies (seaweed)
Beans (red, kidney, pinto, black)
Quinoa
Apple (red, gala, green)
Sweet cherry
Pecan
Prune
Cranberry
Artichokes (cooked)
Turmeric

Coconut oil
Olive oil
Walnuts
Kiwifruit
Soybeans (cooked)
Tofu (raw)
Cauliflower (boiled)
Broccoli (steamed)
Winter squash
Summer squash
Green tea
Papaya and Pineapple
Ginger

Allergy Foods

These 10 allergy foods make up over *90%* of all food allergies. Stay away from them for at least a two weeks and then reintroduce them one at a time to test for sensitivities.

1. Milk
2. Eggs
3. Strawberries
4. Tomatoes
5. Peanuts
6. Tree nuts and butters
7. Soy
8. Fish
9. Shellfish
10. Wheat

Cooking and Eating Rules

~ *preserving the nutrients & enzymes* ~

- The more raw the better, in general.
- Buy small quantities and cook/eat fresh foods (shop at least 2x per week).
- Cook at low temperatures; personally, I never cook above 4 (out of 10) unless I am searing, boiling water or cooking a stew or something similar.
- Do not microwave, fry, smoke, or broil at high temperatures unless you are heating something that is already void of nutrients.
- Plan your meals so you can shop ahead and prepare in advance for 2-4 days at a time.
- Cook with love and attention. Seriously, the food will absorb that energy.
- Use enough oil so things don't stick to the pan, but don't overdo it.
- Make sure your pots and pans are good quality and don't have tears in their lining so the metals leak out.
- Make sure your oils are not old; they will go rancid quicker than you think. Just smell them and you will know. One year is max for most oils, although coconut oil can last 2-5 years.

- Cooking is to activate your foods' enzymes, not make them black or brown. Keep the food crisp and fresh even after cooking.

General EATING RULES

- Organic, cage free, grass fed (not corn fed) and unprocessed
- Chew food into liquid
- Don't eat when stressed or rushed
- Have gratitude for your food
- Small bites helps digestion
- Drink ½ body weight in ounces of water per day
- Get a juicer & juice fruits & vegetables @ least once per month
- Eating fruits in the morning on an empty stomach or by themselves is best
- Eat only one kind of main protein per meal
- DO NOT mix STARCH & PROTEIN, unless you're following food layering rules
- Have *sweets & desserts* by *themselves* as their own meal
- Milk; drink it alone or leave it alone
- Do not eat a lot of fat with proteins

- No cold water w/meals, use 4 ounces max liquid 15 min before or wait until 60 min after meal
- Dried peas, beans, and soybeans; combine mainly with veggies
- Huge meals = waste products
- Follow the 80/20 rules
- Balance yin & yang foods
- Balance alkaline and acidic foods
- Use natural, fermented foods to help digestion; sauerkraut, pickles, vinegar, and more.
- Don't eat within 3 hrs of bedtime

Primary Nutrition

Now it is time to talk about what nutrition really is. What is your definition of nutrition? If you look it up, chances are the definition will be something about food and eating it.

There are two descriptions of nutrition that make sense to me and have changed the way I look at what I eat and, most importantly, how I act.

The first is from **The Integrative Nutrition Institute of New York,** which talks about nutrition coming from two places; food and life. More specifically, they break it down into the following:

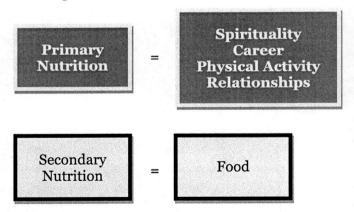

Their philosophy is that if we fill up on primary nutrition, our cravings and need for food, or secondary nutrition, will diminish to more natural urges.

My other favorite definition of nutrition comes from **Dr. Gabriel Cousins,** who explains that nutrition can be thought of as; *all types of energy available to us.*

Dr. Cousins states[1] "...nutrition is what we absorb into our overall body, mind, and spirit from the different density levels that have precipitated from our cosmic force." And he adds that these density levels or energy sources are:

1. Cosmic energy, universal consciousness, God, etc.
2. Sunlight (least dense energy)
3. Oxygen
4. Sexual energy
5. Earths geomagnetic fields
6. Food (most dense energy)

We absorb these energies through various locations (portals) in the body, most importantly[1]:

1. Crown of the head
2. Seven chakras
3. Nose (oxygen)

4. Mouth (food and oxygen)
5. Eyes and skin (sun)
6. Sexual organs
7. Feet or any other part touching the earth (earth's geomagnetic fields)

The functioning efficiency of our energy-receiving areas/portals is directly related to our mental, emotional and spiritual health. Furthermore, the more "in-tune" these components are, the more energy/nutrients we can assimilate into our system.

Because meditation creates harmony within, it has been said that "meditation is the key digestive process through which the life force is taken into the system.[1]"

DON'T WORRY, this is not a philosophical speech! Rather an educational piece on the many possibilities for improving health. If you've made it this far, you are definitely interested in improving your health, and that is what this journey is all about; learning as many different ways to be healthy as possible and choosing which ones feel right for you.

I encourage you to keep an open mind and practice all of these components for at least one month. Our weaknesses often lie in the shadows of our doubts.

Here is a summary of the two definitions of nutrition.

Primary Energy	Secondary Energy
• Sun • Fun • Love • Family • Career • Friends • Oxygen • Sexual energy • Earth's energy • Physical activity • Spirituality/God/etc.	• Food
70-90% Total Energy Source	**10-30% Total Energy Source**

The main issue people face with food and energy comes from focusing on food to fulfill a lack of energy. This lack of energy or hunger for fulfillment is usually stemming from inadequate energy from the primary nutrition components, which leads us to fill up on secondary nutrition, food!

Three keys to reaching an ideal body weight and being healthy are:

1. Making sure our primary nutrition is taken care of
2. Education about eating right
3. Commitment and discipline towards eating to live, not living to eat

Goal # 1 = Increase Primary Nutrition!

Write down three things from *each* energy source (primary and secondary) that you want to work on. Use the examples listed here to get an idea of where you need the most work.

Have fun with this, it can have long lasting effects which encourage new and healthy habits for the future.

Primary	Secondary
• Get outside (sun) • Practice giving hugs, support, etc. for no reason (unconditional love) • Spend more *quality* time with friends or family • Go for meditation walks (earth's energy & exercise) • Abstain from sex for a week in efforts to harness that energy into love • Practice eating less (spiritual) • Focus on your faith and purpose • Mend or end unhealthy relationships • Hiking, walking barefoot, going to the beach, etc. (earth's energy) • Breeaathe (oxygen)	• Carbs/protein/fat *(balance)* • Vitamins and Minerals *(need more)* • Water *(need more)* • Omega 3s *(need more)* • Anti-oxidants *(need more)* • Sugar *(need less)* • Caffeine *(need less)* • Alcohol *(need less)* • Drugs *(need less)* • Red meat or pork *(need less)* • Fruits and veggies *(need more)* • Any other food derivative

Super Alkalizers

These alkalizers really are super, and everyone should have at least two go-to foods. They are your ultimate health enhancers and can be used to combat highly acidic meals and balance the blood.

These meals are alkaline by nature and are ideal for balancing highly acidic meals. **Remember, disease cannot live in an alkaline environment.**

Raw veggies (except for eggplant, asparagus, pickled green olives, Jerusalem artichoke, for example) and salads with natural, unprocessed alkaline dressings

Natural green powder and **probiotic** mixtures. You can find these at health food stores or online

Fresh Juice. If you are serious about your health, then start juicing fresh veggies and fruit ASAP.

Olive oil and Coconut oil

Here are some of my favorite juices;

- *Handful spinach or lettuce, ½ lemon, 1 piece celery, 1 sprig parsley, cucumber sliver, ½ apple, 4 carrots (optional chard and kale leaf)*

- *Handful spinach or lettuce, ½ lemon, 1 piece celery, ¼ of a beet, ½ apple, 3 carrots*

- *½ pear, apple, cucumber and lemon*

On the next page is a good chart to follow for balancing blood acidity levels.

I Balance Blood Acidity by...

Having 2-3 servings of *SUPER ALKALIZERS*...

- Raw veggies or their juices
- Green powders
- Olive or coconut oil

...for every serving of the following *Highly Acidic foods*

- Meats
- Fish/shellfish
- Dairy*
- Cheese*
- Alcohol
- Coffee
- Black teas
- Processed foods
- Sweeteners
- White flour*
- Aspirin
- Tobacco
- Drugs
- Sodas
- Junk food
- Fried foods
- Chocolate*
- Pastries
- Sugars*
- Rice*

*= **processed**

Inflammation Fighters

Here is where food can truly become medicine. Inflammation builds up in us from our food, chemicals, etc. and turns into free radicals that terrorize each blood cell and makes them unable to fight disease and lead to early signs of aging.

While we cannot completely eliminate inflammatory foods from our nutrition plans, we can definitely eliminate and limit some of the unhealthiest, as well as fight them with antioxidant-rich foods.

The best way to keep inflammation down and your blood healthy is to be in *balance* with the foods that cause inflammation. This is also encouraged by following the Yin Yang principles in this Appendix.

Other big factors are:
- How you cook
- Environmental toxins
- Positive attitude
- Anything else that affects your immune system

How to Balance Inflammation with Food

Eat these	Limit these
• Antioxidant foods* • Omega 3s • Green leafy vegetables *See Appendix	• Processed foods • Deep fried foods • Allergy foods* • Night shade vegetables • Wheat and gluten • Rice • White potatoes • Breads • Alcohol • Meats

The No-No List

No matter what the reason, if you are eating any of the following ingredients/additives and you would like to be healthy, please stop consuming them right now. It's that simple. You cannot be healthy if you ***routinely*** consume any of the following 14 items.

I am not going to list the details of why these additives and other toxic ingredients are terrible for you, because if you need to know why you shouldn't have artificial coloring in your blood stream, then you're just not ready yet.

Before we get to the list, check out a few of the problems that the things on The No-No List can cause: i.e., reasons for you and your family to stay away from them.

- Food allergies
- Increased waistlines, obesity and weight gain
- Decreased absorption of minerals and vitamins
- Cancer
- Toxic reactions
- Nervous disorders
- Bloating
- Fatigue

- Arthritis
- Migraines
- Lowered immune function
- Cavities
- Cardiovascular disease
- Osteoporosis
- Depression
- Exaggerated PMS symptoms
- Headaches
- Itchy skin
- Dizziness
- Respiratory issues
- Digestive disorders
- Circulatory dysfunctions
- Coronary problems
- Hyperactivity and ADD in children
- Visual and learning disorders
- Nerve damage
- Liver and kidney damage
- Hair loss
- Behavioral problems
- Fetal abnormalities
- Growth retardation
- Diarrhea and anal leakage
- Heart disease
- Atherosclerosis

- Elevated cholesterol
- Impaired fertility
- Miscarriages and birth defects

Here is The NO-NO LIST....in no particular order. It is up to you to read labels and find out where you are getting them in your diet. The goal is not to be uptight about this list and feel guilty every time you have something on it. The goal is to slowly train your habits so that this list is naturally avoided.

If you eat fresh, whole, organic foods, you won't have to worry about any of this.

The NO-NO LIST

1. Artificial Sweeteners
2. Refined Sugar
3. Pesticides
4. Monosodium Glutamate (MSG)
5. BHA and BHT
6. Sodium Nitrate and Nitrite
7. Soda
8. Artificial Colors
9. Olestra (Olean)
10. Brominated Vegetable Oil (BVO)
11. Partially Hydrogenated Vegetable Oil (Trans Fat)
12. Genetically Modified Organisms (GMOs)
13. High Fructose Corn Syrup (HFCS)
14. Growth hormones in animals

Unrefined vs. Refined Carbs

In studying different cultures around the world from way back when all the way to now, researchers have noticed one main theme: wherever refined carbohydrates are, disease is too.

In short, there are tribes and cultures that eat mainly meat and butter while remaining free from disease and obesity. There are also cultures and tribes that eat mainly starches and vegetarian type foods while staying healthy and free from diseases.

You know what both populations have in common? NO REFINED CARBS. Just natural foods. Every culture that has introduced refined carbohydrates has also introduced diabetes, obesity and heart disease, to name a few problems.

In many ways this is good news because it makes things simple! Just eat natural foods. It doesn't matter if it's meat, butter, potatoes, tomatoes or apples, as long as it's not cake and bread.

Once we alter these sugars as they are found in refined carbohydrates, we take out important ingredients such as fiber, which helps the body process the sugars. Not to mention that they (more the sugars than starch) increase our appetite, are highly addictive and make us eat more than we can burn; an act not seen in nature. Now we have a metabolic mess with these altered sugars that leaves the body full of problems.

Please do your best to get rid of as many refined carbohydrates as possible and only splurge occasionally.

Unrefined Carbohydrates

- Fresh veggies
- Fresh fruits
- Sweet potatoes/yams/potatoes
- Beans and legumes
- Whole grains
- Oatmeal
- Buckwheat
- Amaranth
- Quinoa
- Brown or wild rice
- Basmati rice
- Popcorn
- Raw milk and yogurt (unsweetened)

Refined (Processed) Carbohydrates

- White sugar
- Foods containing corn syrup, HFCS
- Sodas

- Sugary drinks (this includes sweetened fruit juice and tea)
- Alcohol (beer and wine)
- Canned fruits and veggies containing added sugar
- Sweetened applesauce
- White flour and anything made with white flour; bread, muffins, bagels, cakes, cookies, pasta, biscuits, donuts, etc.
- Cereals
- Fries/chips
- Potato chips/pretzels
- Pizza
- Desserts
- White rice
- Boxed puddings
- Candy/toffee/sweets
- Store bought cooked meats/cold cuts (when they have added sugars and additives)
- Sausages/hot dog frankfurters (when they contain carb fillers, additives or sugar)
- Jams/jelly
- Jell-O

Master Cleanse Recipe

Mix the following ingredients together in order to make one master cleanse drink.

- 2 tablespoons of fresh squeezed, organic lemon juice
- 2 tablespoons of organic maple syrup grade B
- 1/10 teaspoon of cayenne pepper powder
- 10 oz distilled water (this is around 295ml of water)

Lemon juice - it will only last for about 8 hours before it turns bad (even if it is refrigerated).

Psyllium Husk Mixture

Psyllium husk is high in fiber and a natural laxative. It helps to facilitate bowel movements and clean out the intestines.

You can find it by itself in a powder-like form or in pre-made cleansing mixtures, such as Perfect. Both work well.

Directions for taking 2x per day

1. Upon waking, take 1-3 teaspoons of psyllium husk with an 8 ounce glass of water. Stir the mixture well, and then drink immediately. Always take psyllium husk with water, otherwise it can expand and interfere with swallowing. Wait for at least 30 minutes before eating a light and healthy breakfast.
2. Drink plenty of water throughout the day and follow the rest of your cleanse guidelines.
3. Take the same mixture of psyllium husk and water before bedtime, on an empty stomach.

Yin & Yang Foods

This list is simply to give you another idea of how to balance your foods. It is common for some people to eat predominantly Yin or Yang. As you can imagine, this violates the very principles of Yin Yang, which is balance.

Yin foods tend to be cooling and/or moistening for the body, while Yang foods tend to be warming and drying. This has less to do with the actual temperature or moisture of the food and more to do with its energy.

The list is too large to fit in this book, so please visit **http://tinyurl.com/7vubbgm** to view the list and see how well you are balancing your food energies.

Coconut Oil

It took me awhile to realize the true benefits of coconut oil and how they differ from person to person.

If you are overweight, lack energy, have poor digestion, high cholesterol and fall into most other categories associated with the average American, then you can experience DRASTIC and life-changing benefits from using coconut oil on a daily basis.

To me, one of the best gifts coconut oil users receive is not directly from the coconut itself. Because coconut oil can replace so many health and beauty products, and even some medications, people will be absorbing 100s to 1000s of less chemicals and man-made "products" every day. That is huge when you read about some of the side effects of these ingredients.

To learn the *Top 40 Reasons to use Coconut Oil,* go here (it will take you to the Cleansing With the Seasons blog) **http://tinyurl.com/4ls29rt**

80/20 Rules

These 80/20 rules are great for obtaining and maintaining health, losing weight, and more. Sometimes other ratios are necessary:

- 90/10 for those who are WAY out of balance and need a boost towards health.
- 60/40 to 80/20 for athletes depending on intensity
- 50/50 to 60/40 for those trying to gain weight

80%	20%
<ul><li>Raw foods</li><li>Healthy & balanced</li><li>Alkaline foods</li><li>Plate of veggies</li><li>Stomach full</li></ul>	<ul><li>Cooked foods</li><li>Eat what you want!!</li><li>Acid foods</li><li>Plate of meat or starches</li><li>Stomach empty</li></ul>

Blood Type Foods

Science* has shown that each of the four blood types, A, B, O and AB, have different capabilities when it comes to breaking down proteins, fats and carbohydrates.

As usual, I didn't believe it until I tried it. But once I did, I realized that my intuitions about many foods were right on. All of the foods that made me congested and bloated were on my "avoid" list for my blood type.

Once I started following the "ideal" and "avoid" foods for my blood type, my health and energy instantly shot up and I had never felt better. And this is coming from someone who already ate healthy, just the wrong healthy foods.

I encourage everyone to give these lists a try and see if you notice any differences. I have yet to have a client that these lists did not work very well for.

You can find all of the lists and many recipes** on the Cleansing With the Seasons blog;
http://seasonalcleansing.wordpress.com/

*The Blood Type Diet is a registered Trademark of Peter J. D'Adamo, N.D., and this book and blog are not affiliated with or sponsored by Dr. D'Adamo.
** These lists, recipes and meal plans are based in part on the work of Peter D'Adamo, N.D.

Bibliography

1. Spiritual Nutrition and The Rainbow Diet. Gabriel Cousins
2. Dr. Stanley Bass (with permission): http://www.drbass.com/sequential.html